The stages of healing and treatment from childhood sexual abuse: A resource guide for a survivor of sexual abuse.

Diego C. Alford

All rights reserved. No part of this publication should be reprinted or transmitted through electronic or mechanical printing without permission from the author.

Copyright © Diego Alfrod, 2022.

Table of content

[Chapter 1](#)
[Chapter 2](#)
[Chapter 3](#)
[Chapter 4](#)

Chapter 1

The gaslighting recovery process

The sexual assault of vulnerable people and children occurs far too frequently throughout the country.

Survivors who encounter this trauma risk a lifetime of emotional challenges and a lower quality of life when they do not actively participate in the healing process. Seeking justice after sexual assault is one of the largest components of healing for survivors. For others, justice is getting their day in court and watching their abuser face the consequences of their acts. This is generally done under the umbrella of criminal justice. Yet, civil action against an abuser also gives a feeling of justice, particularly when too much time has elapsed to file criminal charges.

If you are a victim of sexual abuse, you are not alone. You also need to know learning how to recover from sexual assault is feasible. Many individuals, beginning with family and friends and extending to total strangers, want to support you and empower you as embark on the healing journey.

We have developed this guide to provide you with information on the long-term impact of sexual abuse, how you can recover and rid yourself of some of the effects, and the ways taking legal action with a sexual abuse attorney by your side may assist you with the healing process.

- Why Healing After Surviving Sexual Abuse Is Important.

RAINN (Rape, Abuse & Incest National Network), likely the nation's greatest resource for survivors of sexual abuse and violence, estimates that a perpetrator sexually assaults a child once every nine minutes in the United States. Darkness to Light, a non-profit organization committed to eliminating child sexual abuse, says that child sexual abuse is recognized only about one-third of the time, and victims disclose even less.

This suggests that the majority of persons who underwent sexual abuse throughout their youth are carrying the pain with them while never pursuing any legal action against their abuser.

Oftentimes, survivors ignore thoughts about the abuse and accompanying memories to function in everyday life, and they think it's best to put the past in the past. Yet, putting the trauma deeper might still damage them, particularly if they have specific triggers that bring unresolved anger, resentment, humiliation, and guilt to the surface.

Examples of circumstances that survivors could endure, which lead them to seek aid from others to recover, include:

Uncommon responses to circumstances

Continued challenges with feelings and emotions

Sexual dysfunction

New experiences provoke prior traumas

Survivors of sexual abuse have found that admitting their pain, speaking about it with others, and pursuing justice are crucial components of recovery. Those who participate in the healing process may move beyond their trauma and live healthy lives and remove some or all of the challenges they have had while dealing with their trauma on their own.

Sexual Abuse Recovery
Long-term Impact of Sexual Abuse
Regardless matter the age that a person suffers sexual abuse, the horrific event(s) may damage a victim for years. Child victims of sexual abuse frequently experience the impacts of trauma far into their adult life.
The list below is the most prevalent ways sexual abuse may influence a survivor's life but they can also be

used as symptoms of sexual abuse if you are worried about the well-being of a loved one.

1: Anger and Rage

Some adult survivors of sexual assault describe suffering with rage. In certain scenarios, survivors could be furious with a person, often the abuser, and in other cases, they might be unhappy with a higher authority like their parents, instructors, or caretakers and for enabling them to be abused. Self-hatred is also an outcome of sexual abuse. Survivors feel furious at themselves for their failure to halt the abuse.

2: Depression

Survivors most typically report depression among all the probable long-term effects of sexual abuse. Depression is typically related to post-traumatic stress disorder and comes with several negative symptoms. Those who are depressed frequently suffer from sleeping too little or sleeping too much, changes in appetite, overall unhappiness, and thoughts of despair.

3: Grieving and Mourning

Grieving and sorrow are particularly problematic for adult survivors of childhood sexual abuse. When children endure abuse, they lose innocence and trust, and the capacity to enjoy regular childhood milestones and experiences. If the abuser was a family member, child victims may lose ties with family members or must deal with a shift in relationships.

4: Anxiety, Fear, and Memory

Anyone who undergoes trauma might feel dread and anxiety. Some survivors of childhood sexual abuse retain such dread and worry that they suffer from amnesia or trouble recalling the assault they underwent. Amnesia as a reaction to intense stress happens as a form of survival strategy, particularly for youngsters.

Also, children who were abused at a young age had not yet acquired their communication abilities, thus they were not able to put their experiences and emotions into words. Part of the healing process may entail retrieving repressed memories that some survivors cannot remember.

Chapter 2

How the ghost of your past seems to haunt your present.

Most of us are tormented by the ghosts of our past: that opportunity that we let slip by; that sexual assault or that love interest that treated us horribly and so on.

As we travel through our days we hear our past rattling chains and groaning hauntingly; we see the shadows of our previous errors lurking in the corners, and our past failures sneak up behind us and surprise us at every step. A scared past that is not dealt with generates a fearful future. In addition, to be happy in the present, we need to release the ghosts of the past.

In this article, you'll find 7 strategies to release the ghosts of the past so that you may be happy in the now and the future.

7 Ways to Release the Past
I won't lie to you: shedding the past is hard. Nonetheless, it can be done. Here's what to do:

1. Learn to Live In the Present.

There's no greater way to release the past than to refuse to linger on it. And the greatest approach to abstain from ruminating on the past is to keep your attention firmly focused on the present. When you find yourself thinking about the past, ask yourself the following question:

"Where am I right now?" This will return your focus to the current moment.
The only reason why your history is still bothering you is that you keep it alive in your head by thinking about it. However, if your mind is saturated with the present, there's no place left in it for the past.

2. Change the Past.

If you don't like anything about your history, alter it. Right now you may be thinking: "But it has occurred, there's nothing that I can do to undo it." Although indeed, you can't change what happened in the past, you can change how you interpret the past. Ask yourself questions such as the following:

What happened?
What evidence am I relying on to develop this interpretation?
What assumptions am I making?
Is there another equally credible view of what happened?
How would someone who loves me view this situation?
What's a better, healthier way to perceive this?
I once saw a "Cathy" comic strip in which Cathy's mother bumps across a bunch of ladies she had gone to high school with. The ladies were

exchanging notes about high school, and they informed Cathy's mother that they had always been scared of her because she was gorgeous and received excellent marks. Cathy's mother had always felt that they simply didn't like her.

In the final square of the comic, Cathy's mother says something along the following lines: "All this time I've been building my self-image on the erroneous interpretation." Look for methods to understand the past in a manner that helps you, instead of reading it in ways that damage you.

3. Realize That You're No Longer the Same Person.

Let's imagine that you've always wanted to take up pottery, and you finally decide to attend a class. A few months later you're producing lovely vases, bowls, and so forth. Then you take a look at what you made throughout your first week of class. You'll probably be humiliated by how horrible the things that you generated during that first week are, and you'll want to toss them away.

A lot of the time we assess what we've done in the past through the lens of who we are in the present.

However, our current selves wouldn't behave in the manner we did back then, since we've grown and developed, and we're now wiser. So cut your prior self some slack. As Maya Angelou famously said: "I did then what I knew how to do. Now that I know better, I do better."

4. Let Go Through Ritual.
The human species has been employing rituals from its earliest origins. Create a ritual for a symbolic discharge of poisonous emotions. The sole condition is that the ceremony needs to have significance for you. Fire has long been an element of ritual, and one

ritual you may consider attempting is to write down the tales from the past which are still plaguing you and then burn the piece of paper.

5. Make Room For the New.

One of the finest ways to shed the past is to create a place for the future. What do you do when you're expecting a baby? You empty a room of the home to prepare a nursery. Then, you furnish the nursery with all of the stuff that the baby will require after it's born.

Do the same thing to prepare for your new future. Ask yourself the following:

What type of future do I want?
What does this future require so that it may come into my life?
The future that you desire is on its way. Make a place for it by throwing out all those things from your past that are not in sync with your future vision. In addition, utilize the time and energy that you were devoted to ruminating on the past to accomplish what has to be done to prepare for your vision of the future.

6. Learn to Fail Forward.

For most of us, previous errors have a prominent part in the movies we play in our thoughts. However, instead of assigning our errors the role of adversaries, we may start seeing them as guides that assist and show us the route toward building the future that we desire for ourselves. We can achieve this by learning to fail forward.

Take responsibility for your losses, but don't take failure personally.
View failure as transient.
Have reasonable expectations. A lot of the time we set our expectations so high, that we're setting ourselves

up to fail. Make sure that the objectives that you establish for yourself are reasonable.

Vary your approach. When you fail you've learned something about what doesn't work. Now, try something different.

Learn from your errors and move on.

7. Ask Yourself What You Need to Do To Release The Past.

A while back I acquired a technique called "The Sedona Way", which is simply a method for eliminating unwanted emotions and beliefs. The Sedona Method says that to leave the past you need to ask yourself the following three questions:

Could I let go of this?
Would I let go of this?
If so, when?
When you ask yourself the question, "Could I let go of this?", sometimes the answer will be "no". If this is the case, ask yourself: "What do I need to do to be able to let go of this?" As an illustration, maybe you need to confront someone who's hurt you, or maybe you need to ask forgiveness from someone whom you've harmed in some way.

Chapter 3

Changing patterns

The repercussions of childhood trauma may appear like they can't be healed. But with the appropriate attitude, you may overcome childhood trauma and learn to manage via several stages which include:

1. Recognize the trauma
The adult must accept this distinct childhood event as trauma. It's this initial step of coming to grips with how the tragedy has impacted them and recognizing that it's OK. This will help individuals give meaning to their present issues and make sense of their hardships.

2. Be patient with oneself
Self-criticism and guilt may be particularly frequent when it comes to individuals who have gone

through a difficult upbringing. Some individuals may ask: Why do I behave this way? What's wrong with me? I could have dealt with this in a better manner. These mental processes may lead to despondency and dissatisfaction.

The trick here is to pause and think: you were not responsible for what occurred. Your childhood trauma has left a scar and you're doing your best to recover. But just like any wound, it's crucial to take the time to heal right. Be patient and gentle with yourself. Treat yourself as you would a closest friend.

3. Reach out for assistance
Rely on loved ones for emotional support and understanding. In these circumstances, one of the crucial components is feeling heard, understood, and affirmed. Especially with childhood trauma, one might frequently feel alone and alienated. It's normal to feel that no one will understand or sympathize. But in actuality, this couldn't be further from the truth. If we give individuals the
opportunity, they may become a fantastic support system for us.

The only way to comprehend who we are is to study who we were. This begins with looking at the experiences that have made us into the person we are today. In that process, we will uncover a lot of vital information to work on. It is vital to "normalize" trauma and to be modest enough to work on it with treatment.

In the end, trauma is like a wound that hasn't healed correctly. It requires time, care, attention, and contemplation. No matter what life experiences you might've suffered, it is possible to heal.

Chapter 4

Trusting yourself

Childhood Trauma truly damages trust when people who are meant to love and protect us injure or ignore us instead, trust is shattered. When our caretakers don't reflect our value to us, we never learn to absorb it. We grow up thinking that we don't deserve love, care, and attention.

If our sentiments and emotions are not acknowledged growing up, we come to think that they are invalid, that we shouldn't feel them, and that they are bad. We begin to mistrust ourselves and how we feel. Our sense of trust in our own experience is shaken.

Instead of listening to our inner voice, we allow the outer world to define how to live, feel, and act. We lose a sense of who we are, what we desire, and how we feel. This detachment from our deepest self means that we wind up living a life that isn't truly ours—it's possibly a successful life by contemporary standards, but not a genuine and satisfying one.

This was my experience until I learned to listen to my intuition. Without being able to trust ourselves, we're unable to make judgments, we lack confidence, and we feel like we have no control over our own life. Instead, we are tormented with uncertainty, dread, and self-doubt.

Fortunately, self-trust can be cultivated and increased. Here's what helped me learn to trust my feelings, instincts, and judgment after the trauma of my childhood sexual assault.

Spend time alone and reconnect with yourself.

Carve out some time in the day to simply be and enjoy yourself without any interruptions. This may entail sitting in solitude in your garden, meditating, or simply listening to nature. Maybe you best connect with yourself on lengthy walks. Or maybe you best hear yourself by writing your ideas out—journaling about what is important to you, the lessons you learned from the past, or hopes you have for the future.

Whatever you choose, daily alone time will help you refresh and revitalize, reconnect with who you are, and realign yourself with your actual nature. The idea is to calm your thoughts and create space so that insight may emerge into your consciousness.

Put yourself first

Have your own back and stick up for yourself. Encourage yourself through hard times and appreciate your triumphs. Practice kindness, not perfection.

When I began putting myself first, my entire vibe altered. Instead of turning to others for recognition and acceptance, I searched inside. Instead of waiting for others to please me, I began giving myself the love, care, and attention I desired. By concentrating on addressing my own needs first, I was able to contribute to others from a position of love instead of obligation.

I used to feel nervous, worn out, bitter, and taken for granted. Now I was showing people how I wanted to be treated.

By prioritizing myself, I was conveying a message that my needs are just as essential, and I need love and attention too. The more I showed up for myself, the more I believed that I was worth showing up for. As I established boundaries, abandoned the urge to hang onto toxic or one-sided relationships, and began developing the life I wanted to have, I discovered inner peace. I discovered my value. I came home to myself.

Reclaiming your sense of self and the capacity to trust your instincts and intuition is not only crucial to healing but also establishing a satisfying life.

By reconnecting with myself, practicing mindfulness, resolving trapped energies, and putting myself first, I've learned to access and trust my intuition about what I need and what's best for me. I recovered my value and established a strong sense of self. As a consequence, I no longer attract or accept poisonous relationships or circumstances. I trust that I deserve more and I know you do too.

www.ingramcontent.com/pod-product-compliance
Lightning Source LLC
Chambersburg PA
CBHW050321220526
45465CB00005B/2078